PROSTATE CANCER UNVEILED

'Breaking the Silence, Finding
Hope and Taking Control of Your
Health'

Linda Nwosu, RN

TABLE OF CONTENTS

INTRODUCTION

CHAPTER 1: OVERVIEW OF THE PROSTATE GLAND

1.1 ANATOMY OF THE MALE REPRODUCTIVE SYSTEM

1.2 FUNCTIONS OF THE PROSTATE GLAND

CHAPTER 2: UNDERSTANDING PROSTATE CANCER

2.1 HOW PROSTATE CANCER DEVELOPS

2.2 TYPES OF PROSTATE CANCER

2.3 STAGES OF PROSTATE CANCER

2.4 RISK FACTORS FOR PROSTATE CANCER

2.5 SIGNS AND SYMPTOMS OF PROSTATE CANCER

2.6 IMPORTANCE OF EARLY DETECTION

CHAPTER 3: DIAGNOSIS AND TESTING

3.1 SCREENING FOR PROSTATE CANCER

3.2 DIAGNOSTIC TESTS FOR PROSTATE CANCER

3.3 BIOPSY PROCEDURES AND RESULTS

CHAPTER 4: TREATMENT OPTIONS

4.1 ACTIVE SURVEILLANCE/WATCHFUL WAITING

4.2 SURGERY (PROSTATECTOMY)

4.3 RADIATION THERAPY

4.4 HORMONE THERAPY

4.5 CHEMOTHERAPY

4.6 IMMUNOTHERAPY

CHAPTER 5: COPING WITH PROSTATE CANCER

5.1 EMOTIONAL AND PSYCHOLOGICAL IMPACTS OF PROSTATE CANCER

5.2 COPING STRATEGIES FOR PATIENTS AND CAREGIVERS

5.3 SUPPORT RESOURCES FOR PATIENTS AND FAMILIES

CHAPTER 6: LIVING WITH PROSTATE CANCER

6.1 MANAGING SIDE EFFECTS OF TREATMENT

6.2 FOLLOW-UP CARE AND MONITORING

6.3 LIFESTYLE CHANGES AND PREVENTION
STRATEGIES

CHAPTER 7: FUTURE OF PROSTATE CANCER

7.1 ADVANCES IN RESEARCH AND TREATMENT

7.2 EMERGING THERAPIES AND TECHNOLOGIES

7.3 HOPE FOR A CURE

CONCLUSION

INTRODUCTION

Prostate cancer is the most common cancer among men, with millions of new cases being diagnosed every year. It usually occurs from the ages of 50 years and above, this is because the walnut-shaped gland, the prostate gland, enlarges in size as you advance in age leading to various health challenges. According to the World Cancer Research Fund International, it is the second most commonly occurring cancer in men and the fourth most common cancer generally, and in 2020, there was greater than 1.4 million cases of prostate cancer. Despite its prevalence, the disease remains shrouded in mystery and stigma, leaving many men feeling alone and overwhelmed.

Recently, a popular Nigerian celebrity shared a post on the media about how he conquered prostate cancer, the challenges he faced following the diagnosis and the treatment, and how appreciative he was to have lived through the illness and became a survivor. According to him, it was the biggest fight he has ever had in his life and was elated to have won with the help and support of his loved ones and healthcare providers.

You may think that being diagnosed with this condition is a death sentence. However, it doesn't have to be. With early detection and the right treatment, many men can beat the disease and live full, healthy lives. The key is breaking the silence and taking control of your health. It is important that despite the nature of men and the responsibilities that they shoulder, men should learn to speak up and take actions when necessary regardless of the societal pressures, go for regular check ups as they advance in age, for health is wealth and comes before other necessities of life.

In this book, our goal is to do just that. We will unveil the facts about prostate cancer, starting with helping you understand the anatomy of the male reproductive organ with more emphasis on the prostate gland, exploring the overview of prostate cancer, its causes, symptoms, and treatment options as well as how to cope with the emotional impact of this condition and living through it. We'll also share stories from men who have faced the disease head-on, finding hope and inspiration in their experiences.

Whether you're a man facing a prostate cancer diagnosis or a loved one supporting someone through their journey, this book, **'Prostate Cancer Unveiled: Breaking the Silence, Finding Hope and Taking Control of Your Health'** is for you. We hope it will empower you with the knowledge, tools, and resources you need to take control of your health and find hope in the face of adversity.

CHAPTER 1

OVERVIEW OF THE PROSTATE GLAND

The prostate gland is one of the organs of the male reproductive system. It is about the size of a chest nut and comprises of an apex and a base, an anterior, posterior, and two lateral surfaces. With regards to its location, it is located in front of the rectum, and below the bladder where it surrounds the urethra forming the prostatic urethra. It plays a major role during sexual activity as it produces seminal fluid that aids in the motility of the sperm. It is highly essential that you are equipped with the anatomy of the male reproductive system which would help you understand your physiology, how the various organs work and maintain male reproductive health. Thus, this chapter focuses on discussing this anatomy and the functions of the prostate gland.

1.1 ANATOMY OF THE MALE REPRODUCTIVE SYSTEM

The function of the male reproductive system is to produce, store, and deliver sperm. It consists of several organs, including the testes, epididymis, vas deferens, prostate gland, seminal vesicles, and penis. In this section, we will discuss the anatomy of each of these organs and their functions.

Testes: The testes, or testicles, are the primary male sex organs. The production of sperm and testosterone, the male sex hormone, is dependent on this organ. The testes are located in the scrotum, a pouch of skin that hangs below the penis. The scrotum aids in the regulation of the temperature of the testes, which is vital for sperm production.

Epididymis: This is a long, coiled tube that is located on the back of each testicle. It is responsible for storing and transporting sperm from the testes to the vas deferens. During this process, the sperm mature and become more mobile.

Vas Deferens: The vas deferens serves as a passageway. It is a muscular tube that helps in the carriage of sperm from the epididymis to the urethra. It is about 18 inches long and travels through the spermatic cord, a bundle of nerves, blood vessels, and other tissues that run from the testes to the abdominal cavity.

Prostate Gland: The prostate gland is a walnut-sized gland that sits just below the bladder. It is responsible for producing some of the fluids that make up semen. The prostate gland also helps to control the flow of urine by surrounding the urethra, the tube that carries urine and semen out of the body.

Seminal Vesicles: These are two miniature glands situated behind the bladder. They produce a fluid that makes up a significant portion of semen. The fluid contains nutrients that help to nourish and protect the sperm.

Penis: The penis is located externally. It is the external male sex organ. It is composed of three parts: the root, shaft, and glans. The root of the penis attaches it to the pelvic bone. The shaft is the long, cylindrical part of the penis. The glans is the vascular body that forms the apex of the penis. During sexual arousal, there is blood flow into the penis, causing erection. This allows for penetration and ejaculation during sexual intercourse.

1.2 FUNCTIONS OF THE PROSTATE GLAND

The most essential function of the prostate gland is the production of semen. It creates an alkaline fluid that mixes with the sperm during ejaculation to form semen. This fluid helps in nourishing and protecting the sperm once it gets to the vagina which is an acidic environment.

In addition, the muscles of these gland ensures that this fluid is squeezed into the urethra and expelled with sperm as semen during ejaculation.

Another function of the prostate gland is the production of hormones. In the prostate, the male hormone, testosterone is metabolized to a biologically active form known as Dihydrotestosterone (DHT). This hormone, DHT is responsible for the male sex drive and this can reduce with age advancement.

It produces Prostate-Specific Antigen (PSA). This fluid acts as a glue, hence, helping the sperm to attach to the woman's cervix. This glue dissolves eventually, allowing the sperm to swim freely into the uterus to find an egg. High levels of this antigen is an indication of prostate cancer. Therefore, it is advisable that men beyond the ages of 50 check their PSA levels annually which is done through a simple blood test. The gland also helps in urine flow regulation. During ejaculation, it ensures that no urine is mixed with sperm.

CHAPTER 2

UNDERSTANDING PROSTATE CANCER

Cancer results when there is an abnormal growth of cells taking over the normal cell function, making it difficult for the body to work effectively. Therefore, prostate cancer refers to the formation and growth of abnormal cells in the prostate gland. Prostate cancer is the second most commonly diagnosed cancer in men and ranks fourth in the prevalent cancers diagnosed worldwide. It is estimated that one in eight men will develop prostate cancer at some point in their life and majority of these cases are usually diagnosed in men aged 65 years and above. When this cancer is at the local or regional stage, that is, within the prostate, it is highly treatable and there is a higher chance of survival compared to when it has metastasized to other organs which can be life threatening.

2.1 HOW PROSTATE CANCER DEVELOPS

Prostate cancer is a type of cancer that occurs in the prostate gland, a small gland which is a component of the male reproductive system. The prostate gland is responsible for producing the fluid that nourishes and transports sperm during ejaculation. Prostate cancer is one of the most common types of cancer in men and typically develops slowly over many years.

Although the exact pathophysiology of prostate cancer is not fully understood yet, it is believed that the development of prostate cancer begins when cells in the prostate gland start to grow and divide uncontrollably. This uncontrolled growth leads to the formation of a tumor. In the early stages of prostate cancer, the tumor is usually confined to the prostate gland and may not cause any noticeable symptoms.

As the tumor grows, it can put pressure on the urethra, which is the tube that carries urine from the bladder out of the body. This can cause symptoms such as difficulty urinating, urinating frequently, and inability to sustain a urine stream. These symptoms are often a sign that the cancer has grown beyond the prostate gland and may have spread to nearby tissues.

Prostate cancer can also spread to other parts of the body through a process called metastasis. Cancer cells can break away from the tumor and enter the bloodstream or lymphatic system, which can carry them to other parts of the body. The most common sites of metastasis for prostate cancer are the bones and lymph nodes.

The exact cause of prostate cancer is not fully comprehended, but several risk factors have been identified. Age is the most significant risk factor, with the incidence of prostate cancer increasing significantly after the age of 50. Other risk factors include a family history of prostate cancer, a diet high in fat and low in fruits and vegetables, red meats and diary products and exposure to certain chemicals.

2.2 TYPES OF PROSTATE CANCER

Although prostate cancer develops when there is uncontrollable growth of abnormal cells in the prostate, not all abnormal growths also referred to as tumors are cancerous in nature. While some are malignant, that is cancerous, certain tumors are not. (benign).

There are several types of prostate cancer, each with unique characteristics and behaviors, depending on the type of cell they started in. Understanding the different types of prostate cancer is crucial in determining the most effective treatment plan. The following are the most common types of prostate cancer:

Adenocarcinoma: This type of prostate cancer is the most common and accounts for over 95% of all cases. Adenocarcinoma starts in the glandular cells of the prostate gland, these cells produce the prostate fluid and grows slowly over time. It is usually confined to the prostate gland and may not cause any symptoms.

Small cell carcinoma: This type of prostate cancer is rare and accounts for less than 1% of all cases. Small cell carcinoma starts in the neuroendocrine cells of the prostate gland and grows rapidly. It is aggressive and can spread quickly to other parts of the body compared to other types of prostate cancer.

Sarcomas: Sarcomas are rare types of prostate cancer that start in the connective tissues of the prostate gland. These cancers are usually aggressive and tend to spread quickly to other parts of the body.

Transitional cell carcinoma: Transitional cell carcinoma starts in the cells that line the urethra, which is the tube that carries urine out of the body. It usually starts in the bladder and spreads to the prostate. This type of prostate cancer is rare accounting between 2 and 4% out of 100 prostate cancers and can be aggressive.

Ductal adenocarcinoma: Ductal adenocarcinoma begins in the cells that line the prostate gland ducts. This type of cancer is rare and aggressive, and can spread to other parts of the body.

2.3 STAGES OF PROSTATE CANCER

The stages of prostate cancer are majorly grouped into four beginning with the early stage.

Prostate cancer can be divided into several stages, which are used to determine the severity of the disease and the appropriate course of treatment. In this section, we will discuss the different stages of prostate cancer and their characteristics.

Stage 1: In stage 1 prostate cancer, the cancer is small and confined to the prostate gland. It is usually detected during a routine checkup, and often does not cause any symptoms. Treatment for stage 1 prostate cancer may include active surveillance, which involves monitoring the cancer through regular checkups and imaging tests, or treatment with surgery or radiation therapy.

Stage 2: In stage 2 prostate cancer, the cancer has grown beyond the prostate gland but has not spread to other parts of the body. It may be detected through a prostate-specific antigen (PSA) blood test or a digital rectal exam. Treatment for stage 2 prostate cancer may include surgery, radiation therapy, or a combination of both.

The Stage 1 and 2 are often called the **'early-stage'** or **'localized'** prostate cancer as it is still within the confines of the prostate gland.

Stage 3: In stage 3 prostate cancer, the cancer has spread beyond the prostate gland and may have invaded nearby tissues, such as the seminal vesicles or the bladder. It may also have spread to nearby lymph nodes and commonly called **'locally-advanced prostate cancer'** . Treatment may include surgery, radiation therapy, or hormone therapy, which is used to decrease the level of testosterone in the body and slow the growth of cancer cells.

Stage 4: In stage 4 prostate cancer, the cancer has spread to other parts of the body, such as the bones, liver, or lungs. This is termed **metastatic or advanced prostate cancer**. Treatment for stage 4 prostate cancer may include hormone therapy, chemotherapy, radiation therapy, or a combination of these treatments.

2.4 RISK FACTORS FOR PROSTATE CANCER

The actual cause of prostate cancer is idiopathic. However, there are certain factors that can predispose a man to this disease.

Age: As a man advances in age, the prostate gland tends to enlarge. This increase a man's risk of developing this condition, with most cases being diagnosed in men over the ages of 65.

Family history: Men with a family history of prostate cancer, are at a higher chance of developing the disease themselves. Also, having family members with a history of ovarian and breast cancer increases the chances of having this condition.

Ethnicity: Amongst other ethnicities, African-American men are at a higher risk of developing prostate cancer. It is estimated that one in six men from this race will be diagnosed with prostate cancer.

Weight: Research has shown that being overweight in your 50's raises the risk of prostate cancer. Therefore, it is advisable to maintain a healthy body mass index.

Diet: A diet rich in red meat and dairy products may elevate the risk of prostate cancer.

2.5 SIGNS AND SYMPTOMS OF PROSTATE CANCER

It is important to note that the symptoms of prostate cancer may not appear until the disease has progressed to later stages. As the cancer progresses, however, the following signs and symptoms may occur:

- Difficulty urinating
- Weak or interrupted urine flow
- Painful urination
- Blood in the urine or semen
- Frequent urination in the night (nocturia)
- Painful ejaculation
- Regular pain mostly in the lower back, hips, or upper thighs

2.6 THE IMPORTANCE OF EARLY DETECTION

As men age, the prostate gland can enlarge, leading to a condition known as benign prostatic hyperplasia (BPH). While BPH is not cancerous, it can cause symptoms such as difficulty urinating, frequent urination, and a weak urine stream.

Early-stage prostate cancer often does not cause any symptoms, which is why regular check ups and routine screening is so important. Screening for prostate cancer typically involves a blood test known as the prostate-specific antigen (PSA) test and a digital rectal exam (DRE). If prostate cancer is suspected, a biopsy may be performed to confirm the diagnosis. These actions are critical for successful outcomes which can only be established at the early stages of the prostate cancer. Detecting prostate cancer at the initial stage is a win-win because it helps to increase the chances of survival on the individual, reduces the financial and emotional stress placed on the patients and their families as well as reduces the pressure on health facilities. Therefore, it is important that men are well informed that check ups should be carried out regularly as they get older to decrease the rate of mortality from prostate cancer.

CHAPTER 3

DIAGNOSIS AND TESTING

Prostate cancer is a common type of cancer that affects men, with an estimated 248,530 new cases diagnosed in the United States in 2021 alone. Fortunately, prostate cancer can often be detected early through screening tests, allowing for earlier treatment and improved outcomes. Prostate cancer is typically diagnosed through a combination of a physical exam, blood tests, and a biopsy of the prostate gland. During a physical exam, a healthcare provider may feel for any abnormalities in the prostate gland. Blood tests can measure levels of prostate-specific antigen (PSA), which may be elevated in men with prostate cancer. A biopsy involves taking a small sample of tissue from the prostate gland to be examined under a microscope.

3.1 SCREENING FOR PROSTATE CANCER

The two primary screening tests for prostate cancer are the prostate-specific antigen (PSA) blood test and the digital rectal exam (DRE).

The PSA test helps in the measurement of the level of PSA in the blood, which is a protein manufactured by the prostate gland. Elevated PSA levels may indicate the presence of prostate cancer, although other factors such as age, race, certain medical conditions such as benign prostate hyperplasia which is a non-cancerous enlargement of the prostate as men age, and certain medications can also affect PSA levels. If the PSA test is abnormal, a prostate biopsy may be suggested to determine if you really have cancer. The PSA levels in the blood is measured in the units known as **nanograms per milliliter (ng/ml)**. Most medical practitioners use a cut off point of 4 ng/ml in diagnosing this condition, however, a range less than 4 ng/ml does not mean that one doesn't have cancer. Men having a PSA level between 4 and 10 ng/mL commonly called **'the borderline range'** have 1 in 4 chance of having this condition and a level above 10 increases the chances to greater than 50%.

The American Cancer Society recommends that men discuss the potential benefits and risks of PSA testing with their healthcare provider starting at age 50, or at age 45 for men at a greater risk (such as African American men or men with a genetic history of prostate cancer).

The DRE involves a healthcare provider inserting a gloved finger into the rectum to feel the prostate gland for any abnormalities or lumps. While the DRE can be uncomfortable, it is a relatively simple and quick procedure that can help detect prostate cancer in its early stages.

3.2 DIAGNOSTIC TESTS FOR PROSTATE CANCER

If screening tests suggest the presence of prostate cancer, diagnostic tests such as a biopsy may be necessary to confirm the diagnosis. During a biopsy, a small sample of prostate tissue is removed and examined under a microscope for the presence of cancerous cells.

Imaging tests such as a prostate MRI or a CT scan may also be used to help diagnose prostate cancer or determine the extent of the cancer.

After a diagnosis of prostate cancer is confirmed, staging tests may be performed to determine the extent of the cancer and whether it has spread to other parts of the body. Staging tests may include imaging tests such as bone scans, CT scans, or MRI scans.

3.3 BIOPSY PROCEDURES AND RESULTS

A biopsy is a medical procedure that involves collection of a small snippet of tissue from the body. This tissue can be examined under a microscope to look for signs of disease. In the case of prostate cancer biopsy, a thin needle is used to collect samples of tissue from the prostate and then viewed under a microscope to detect cancer. This may be performed to confirm a diagnosis, determine the severity of the cancer, or monitor the progression of the disease.

Prostate biopsy has some advantages as it is a definite diagnosis for prostate cancer, helps in early detection of prostate cancer and determines how quickly it can metastasize, nevertheless, it has certain disadvantages such as side effects like infections, pain and short term bleeding. However, the benefits outweigh the risks in this condition and you will be informed of this before the procedure by your health care provider in order to make an informed decision. There are two major types of prostate biopsy which includes, trans-rectal ultrasound (TRUS) guided biopsy and trans-perineal biopsy.

The trans-rectal ultrasound (TRUS) guided biopsy is the most common and is typically performed on an outpatient basis. It involves the passage of the needle through the wall of the rectum to collect small sample tissues from the prostate. During this procedure, you will maintain a knee-chest position while an ultrasound probe is inserted into your rectum. This is made less discomforting by the application of a gel and the administration of a local anesthetic which numbs the area around your prostate. This ultrasound probe scans the prostate and displays the image on a screen guiding the health practitioner on the area to collect samples from. After the application of a local anesthetic, a needle is placed next to the probe through the rectum and into your prostate and about 10 to 12 tiny pieces of tissues are collected from different areas of the prostate, but this can be made fewer by images from an MRI scan. This process usually takes about 5 to 10 minutes and after the procedure, your doctor would ensure that you can pass urine as one of the side effect of biopsy is acute urinary retention as biopsy causes the prostrate to increase in size.

The trans-perineal biopsy is less common but may be used in certain cases. It involves the insertion of the biopsy needle into the prostate through the skin between the scrotum and the anus. It can be done either under a general or local anesthesia. It is of two types which includes, the targeted or template trans-perineal biopsy.

Results of a Biopsy

After a biopsy, the tissue samples will be sent to a laboratory for analysis. A pathologist will examine the tissue under a microscope to look for signs of cancer. The results of a biopsy may include:

Negative: If no cancer cells are found in the tissue samples, the biopsy is considered negative. However, a negative biopsy does not necessarily mean that cancer is not present. If a man has a high level of suspicion for prostate cancer based on other factors, further testing may be necessary.

Positive: If cancer cells are found in the tissue samples, the biopsy is considered positive. The pathologist will also assign a Gleason score, which is a measure of how aggressive the cancer is based on the appearance of the cancer cells under the microscope.

Inconclusive: In some cases, the tissue samples may not provide a clear answer. This can occur if the biopsy samples do not contain enough tissue or if the tissue samples are not of high enough quality to make a definitive diagnosis. In these cases, additional testing may be necessary.

Biopsy procedures for prostate cancer are an important tool for diagnosing and monitoring the disease. If you are at risk for prostate cancer or have symptoms, it is crucial to talk to your healthcare provider about whether a biopsy may be appropriate for you. Remember, early detection and treatment can increase the chances of a successful outcome.

CHAPTER 4

TREATMENT OPTIONS

Treatment for prostate cancer depends on several factors, including the stage and grade of the cancer, the patient's age and overall health, and the patient's personal preferences. Treatment options may include surgery, radiation therapy, hormone therapy, chemotherapy, immunotherapy, and active surveillance/watchful waiting. Choosing a treatment option for this disease condition can be a herculean task. Most prostate cancer survivors in their stories shared that one of the difficult decisions they ever made after being diagnosed of prostate cancer was choosing a treatment option. Although they were skeptical about their choices, they believed it was the best for them after weighing its benefits and risks from the appropriate information given to them by their healthcare provider. According to American Cancer Society, a prostate cancer survivor, Brian Glennon, while sharing his story after the diagnosis and making his treatment decisions said, " Sometimes, of course, we are not sure of what to do at times like this. Certain individuals like to reach out, others like to render assistance, some people are fearful they will say the wrong thing, and some people cope much better with going about their day-to-day routines. My advice is simple- do whatever makes you feel comfortable ''. So, I hope you choose whatever treatment option that makes you feel comfortable and which you are willing to take the risks. In this chapter, we would be exploring some of the treatment options which would help you stay informed of what each entails.

4.1 ACTIVE SURVEILLANCE/ WATCHFUL WAITING

In certain cases, doctors may recommend monitoring the cancer closely to see if it progresses before deciding on treatment. Active surveillance and watchful waiting are two strategies used to manage prostate cancer. These approaches are often recommended for men with low-risk or early-stage prostate cancer.

Active surveillance involves closely monitoring the cancer through regular prostate-specific antigen (PSA) tests, digital rectal exams (DREs), and periodic biopsies. If the cancer shows signs of progression such as an increase in PSA levels or changes in the size or shape of the prostate gland, then treatment may be recommended.

Watchful waiting, on the other hand, involves monitoring the cancer but not actively treating it. This approach is typically reserved for men who have a limited life expectancy or other health problems that make treatment risky or impractical.

Both active surveillance and watchful waiting can help avoid the potential side effects and complications of more aggressive treatments like surgery or radiation therapy. However, they also require a high level of patient engagement and compliance with monitoring protocols.

It's important to note that active surveillance and watchful waiting are not interchangeable terms. Active surveillance involves a more active approach to monitoring the cancer and may involve more frequent testing and biopsies. Watchful waiting, on the other hand, is a more passive approach that may involve less frequent testing and monitoring. If you are considering active surveillance or watchful waiting for prostate cancer, it's important to discuss the pros and cons of these approaches with your healthcare provider. Factors that may influence the decision include your age, overall health, and the stage and grade of your cancer.

In some cases, your healthcare provider may recommend combining active surveillance or watchful waiting with other interventions, such as lifestyle changes or targeted therapies, to help slow the progression of the cancer.

Regardless of the approach you choose, it's important to stay engaged in your care and to work closely with your healthcare provider to monitor the cancer and make informed decisions about treatment. With the right approach and support, active surveillance and watchful waiting can be effective strategies for managing prostate cancer and improving quality of life.

4.2 SURGERY (PROSTATECTOMY)

Prostatectomy is a surgical procedure performed to remove the prostate gland, which is located just below the bladder in men. It may be recommended for some patients, especially those with early-stage prostate cancer.

The most common reason for a prostatectomy is prostate cancer, which is one of the prevalent types of cancer in men. Other reasons include an enlarged prostate, which can cause urinary problems, and prostatitis, which is an inflammation of the prostate gland.

There are two main types of prostatectomy: radical prostatectomy and simple prostatectomy. Radical prostatectomy is the most common type of prostatectomy and involves the removal of the entire prostate gland, as well as the seminal vesicles and sometimes nearby lymph nodes. Simple prostatectomy is a less invasive procedure that only removes a portion of the prostate gland.

Prostatectomy can be performed using several different surgical techniques which can be either open surgery, laparoscopic or robot-assisted surgery. Open surgery involves making a large incision in the abdomen or perineum to access the prostate gland. Laparoscopic surgery is a minimally invasive technique that uses small incisions and a camera to guide the surgeon's instruments. Robot-assisted surgery is a type of laparoscopic surgery that uses a robotic system to perform the surgery.

After prostatectomy, patients may experience side effects such as urinary incontinence, erectile dysfunction, and changes in ejaculation. However, many of these side effects can be managed with medications or other treatments.

It is important for patients to discuss the risks and benefits of prostatectomy with their healthcare provider before deciding on this procedure. Additionally, patients should follow all post-operative instructions and attend follow-up appointments to ensure a smooth recovery.

4.3 RADIATION THERAPY

Radiation therapy is a common treatment option for prostate cancer. It works by using high-energy radiation to kill cancer cells in the prostate gland and may be used to treat both early-stage and advanced prostate cancer. This radiation can be delivered either externally or internally. External beam radiation therapy involves the use of a machine that directs radiation from outside the body towards the prostate gland while Internal radiation therapy, also known as brachytherapy, involves the positioning of radioactive seeds within the prostate gland. This therapy may be used alone or in combination with other treatments, such as surgery or hormone therapy. The choice of treatment depends on several factors, including the stage and grade of the cancer, the age and overall health of the patient, and the patient's personal preferences.

One advantage of radiation therapy is that it is a non-invasive treatment option that does not require surgery. This means that there is no surgical incision, and the recovery time is generally shorter than that of surgery. Additionally, radiation therapy can be delivered on an outpatient basis, meaning that patients can go home the same day and continue with their daily activities. However, radiation therapy does have some potential side effects. These can include fatigue, urinary and bowel problems, and sexual dysfunction. Most of these side effects are temporary and can be managed with medication and lifestyle modifications. It is very uncommon for radiation therapy to cause long-term side effects, such as damage to surrounding organs or tissues.

To minimize the risk of side effects, radiation therapy is carefully planned and monitored by a team of healthcare professionals, including a radiation oncologist, a medical physicist, and a radiation therapist. The radiation oncologist will work with the patient to develop an individualized treatment plan that takes into account the patient's unique circumstances and needs.

Overall, radiation therapy is a safe and effective treatment option for prostate cancer that can help to control or cure the disease. It is important that you speak with your healthcare provider to learn more about the   benefits and risks of radiation therapy and to determine if it is the right treatment option for you.

4.4 HORMONE THERAPY

Hormone therapy may be used to lower the levels of hormones that can cause prostate cancer to grow. It is a treatment option that is often used to slow the growth of prostate cancer.

The growth and division of prostate cancer cells is dependent on the male hormone, testosterone. This hormone therapy works by blocking the production or action of testosterone in the body.

Types of Hormone Therapy

There are several types of hormone therapy that can be used to treat prostate cancer, including:

Luteinizing hormone-releasing hormone (LHRH) agonists: These drugs stop the production of testosterone in the testicles by blocking the signal from the brain to the testicles to produce testosterone. Examples of these drugs include leuprolide, goserelin, and triptorelin.

Anti-androgens: These drugs block the action of testosterone in the body by preventing it from binding to the androgen receptor on prostate cancer cells. Examples of these drugs include bicalutamide, flutamide, and nilutamide.

Orchiectomy: This surgical procedure removes the testicles, which are the main source of testosterone in men. It is usually reserved for men who cannot or do not wish to take medications.

Combined androgen blockade (CAB): This involves using both an LHRH agonist and an anti-androgen to block testosterone production and action.

Estrogen therapy: This is rarely used now due to the risk of serious side effects, but it was once a common treatment for advanced prostate cancer.

Side Effects of Hormone therapy

Hormone therapy can cause a range of side effects, including, hot flashes and night sweats, loss of libido, erectile dysfunction, breast enlargement and tenderness, fatigue, weight gain, anemia, osteoporosis, depression, memory and concentration problems.

Hormone therapy is a valuable treatment option for prostate cancer that has spread beyond the prostate gland or has recurred after initial treatment. However, it can cause significant side effects, so it is important for men to discuss the risks and benefits of hormone therapy with their healthcare provider before starting treatment. Regular monitoring and follow-up appointments with a healthcare provider can help manage any side effects and ensure the treatment is working effectively.

4.5 CHEMOTHERAPY

While many prostate cancers are slow-growing and do not require treatment, some can be more aggressive and may require chemotherapy as part of the treatment plan.

What is chemotherapy?

Chemotherapy is a type of cancer treatment that utilizes drugs to cause destruction of the cancer cells. Chemotherapy drugs are designed to target rapidly dividing cells, which cancer cells are. The drugs can be given intravenously, through a pill, or injected into a muscle. Depending on the type of cancer and the stage of the disease, chemotherapy may be used alone or in combination with other treatments like surgery, radiation therapy, or hormone therapy.

How is chemotherapy used to treat prostate cancer?

Chemotherapy is not typically the first line of treatment for prostate cancer. Instead, it is usually reserved for cases where the cancer has spread beyond the prostate gland or is not responding to other treatments. Chemotherapy may also be used in combination with hormone therapy to slow the growth of cancer cells.

The most common chemotherapy drugs used for prostate cancer are docetaxel and cabazitaxel. These drugs work by preventing cancer cells from dividing and multiplying. They are usually given in cycles, with a period of rest in between to allow the body to recover.

Chemotherapy may also be used as a palliative treatment to relieve symptoms in men with advanced prostate cancer. This type of chemotherapy may help shrink tumors, reduce pain, and improve overall quality of life.

What are the potential side effects of chemotherapy for prostate cancer?

Chemotherapy drugs can affect healthy cells in addition to cancer cells, which can lead to side effects. Some of the most common side effects of chemotherapy for prostate cancer include:

- Fatigue
- Nausea and vomiting
- Hair loss
- Loss of appetite
- Diarrhea
- Increased risk of infection
- Anemia (low red blood cell count)
- Easy bruising or bleeding
- Peripheral neuropathy (numbness or tingling in hands or feet)

Most side effects of chemotherapy are temporary and will go away after treatment is complete. However, some side effects, such as peripheral neuropathy, may be long-lasting.

Conclusively, chemotherapy is a type of cancer treatment that can be used to treat prostate cancer in certain cases. While it can be an effective treatment, it is not without side effects. If you or someone you know is considering chemotherapy for prostate cancer, be sure to discuss the potential benefits and risks with a healthcare provider.

4.6 IMMUNOTHERAPY

Prostate cancer is one of the most common types of cancer in men worldwide. While treatments such as surgery, radiation therapy, and chemotherapy have been used to manage this disease, there is increasing interest in the use of immunotherapy as a potential treatment option. Immunotherapy works by enabling the stimulation of the immune system to detect and fight cancer cells.

What is Immunotherapy?

Immunotherapy is a type of cancer treatment that makes use of the body's immune system to destroy cancer cells. The immune system is responsible for detecting and destroying foreign invaders such as viruses and bacteria, as well as abnormal cells, including cancer cells. However, cancer cells can often evade detection by the immune system, allowing them to continue to grow and spread. In order to overcome this, immunotherapy focuses on boosting the ability of the immune system to recognize and attack cancer cells.

Types of Immunotherapy

There are various types of immunotherapy, including:

Immune checkpoint inhibitors: These drugs target proteins on immune cells that prevent them from attacking cancer cells. By blocking these proteins, immune checkpoint inhibitors can help the immune system recognize and attack cancer cells more effectively.

CAR T-cell therapy: This is a type of immunotherapy that involves removing T cells from a patient's blood and genetically modifying them to recognize and attack cancer cells. These modified cells are then infused back into the patient's body, where they can seek out and destroy cancer cells.

Cancer vaccines: These vaccines are structured to induce the immune system to recognize and attack cancer cells.

They can be made from cancer cells themselves, or from specific proteins or other molecules found on cancer cells.

Immunotherapy for Prostate Cancer

Several immunotherapy treatments have been developed specifically for prostate cancer. One of the most promising is immune checkpoint inhibitors, which have shown promising results in clinical trials. In particular, a drug called pembrolizumab has been shown to improve survival in patients with advanced prostate cancer.

Another potential treatment is CAR T-cell therapy, which is currently being studied in clinical trials. This approach involves genetically modifying a patient's T cells to recognize and attack prostate cancer cells.

Finally, cancer vaccines are also being developed for prostate cancer. These vaccines can be made from proteins found on prostate cancer cells, or from other molecules that are specific to prostate cancer.

Side Effects

Similar to other cancer treatments, immunotherapy has certain side effects. These can include fatigue, fever, nausea, and muscle aches. However, immunotherapy tends to cause fewer side effects than traditional chemotherapy, and the side effects are generally less severe.

Overall, Immunotherapy is a promising new approach to the treatment of prostate cancer. While more research is needed to determine the best ways to use immunotherapy in the management of this disease, early results suggest that it could be an effective treatment option for some patients. If you or a loved one has been diagnosed with prostate cancer, it's important to talk to your doctor about all of the available treatment options, including immunotherapy.

CHAPTER 5

COPING WITH PROSTATE CANCER

John had always been active and maintained a healthy lifestyle. He had taken good care of himself, eating well and exercising regularly. However, as he approached his 50th birthday, he started to notice some changes in his body that he couldn't ignore.

At first, he didn't think much of it. He attributed the frequent urination to his age and the occasional pain during urination to a urinary tract infection. But when the symptoms persisted, he knew he needed to see a doctor.

John made an appointment with his primary care physician and explained his symptoms. His doctor recommended he undergo some tests, including a digital rectal exam and a prostate-specific antigen (PSA) test.

John was nervous about the tests but he knew it was necessary to get to the bottom of what was causing his symptoms. During the digital rectal exam, his doctor felt a lump on his prostate, which was concerning. The PSA test also came back with a high level, which further indicated that something was not right.

His doctor referred him to a specialist for further evaluation. The specialist performed a biopsy of the prostate, and a few days later, John received the devastating news that he had prostate cancer.

John was shocked and scared. He had never expected to hear those words, and he didn't know what to do next. The specialist explained the treatment options available to him, including surgery, radiation, and chemotherapy.

After discussing the pros and cons of each option with his doctors and loved ones, John decided to undergo surgery to remove the cancerous prostate. The surgery was successful, and John's doctors were hopeful that they caught the cancer early enough that it hadn't spread beyond the prostate.

John had a long road to recovery ahead of him, but he was grateful for the early diagnosis and the swift action taken by his doctors. He knew that he had a tough road ahead of him, but he was determined to beat the cancer and return to a healthy and active lifestyle.

Just like John, hearing this diagnosis can be a shocking news and may take some time to absorb. It doesn't only affect you but others around you, your families and friends, however, how you handle and cope with this condition matters. In this chapter, we would be discussing how to deal with the emotional impact of this condition, coping strategies and support resources for patients and their families.

5.1 EMOTIONAL AND PSYCHOLOGICAL IMPACTS OF PROSTATE CANCER

At the point of diagnosis of this condition, you really might not know what to do next or how to absorb the news just like John. Asides the physiological effects of prostate cancer which are well-known, it has emotional and psychological impacts which are often overlooked and if not handled effectively can cause more damage than the condition itself. Dealing with prostate cancer can be overwhelming and beating it is dependent on the mindset which would allow you focus on the treatment options and adhere to them while being hopeful on the outcome. The emotional impact of prostate cancer ranges from fear and anxiety to depression and anger.

Fear and Anxiety

One of the most common emotions men experience after a prostate cancer diagnosis is fear. Fear of the unknown, fear of treatment, and fear of the cancer spreading can be overwhelming. Anxiety is also common and can be caused by the stress of the diagnosis, treatment, and the uncertainty of the future.

To manage fear and anxiety, it is important to talk to your doctor or a mental health professional. They can help you understand your diagnosis, discuss your treatment options, and provide you with coping strategies. Mindfulness meditation, deep breathing exercises, and other relaxation techniques can also help you manage anxiety.

Depression

Depression is another common emotional response to a prostate cancer diagnosis. The stress of the diagnosis, treatment, and changes to your life can take a toll on your mental health. Depression can cause a range of symptoms, including sadness, fatigue, changes in appetite, and difficulty sleeping.

If you are feeling depressed, it is essential to seek help. Talking to a mental health professional or joining a support group can be beneficial. Exercise, spending time with loved ones, and engaging in hobbies or other activities you enjoy can also help improve your mood.

Anger

Anger is a natural response to a prostate cancer diagnosis. You may feel angry that you have been diagnosed with cancer, or angry at the changes in your life that the diagnosis brings. It is pertinent to acknowledge these feelings of anger and discover healthy ways to express them.

Talking to a mental health professional or joining a support group can provide a safe space to express your anger. Exercise, writing in a journal, and practicing relaxation techniques can also help you manage your anger.

5.2 COPING STRATEGIES FOR PATIENTS AND CAREGIVERS.

Prostate cancer is a challenging diagnosis for both patients and their caregivers. Coping with the physical and emotional effects of this disease can be overwhelming. In addition to seeking professional help, there are strategies that can help you and your caregivers manage the stress and improve the quality of life.

Here are some coping strategies for patients with prostate cancer and their caregivers:

Staying informed: Educating yourself about your diagnosis, treatment options, and the potential side effects can help you and your caregivers feel more in control.

Building a support network: Friends, family, and support groups can provide emotional support and practical help. It is important to solicit support from relatives, friends, and healthcare providers. Joining a support group can also provide a safe space to discuss and share experiences with others who are going through the same challenges.

Practicing self-care: Eating a healthy diet, exercising regularly, getting enough sleep, and reducing stress can help improve your physical and mental health. It may also help to reduce the risk of recurrence.

Communication: Communication is key to understanding and addressing the patient's needs. Patients should feel comfortable discussing their symptoms, side effects of treatment, and concerns with their healthcare provider, family, and caregivers.

Manage Side Effects: Prostate cancer treatment can cause side effects such as fatigue, pain, and urinary incontinence. Patients and caregivers should work with their healthcare providers to manage these side effects effectively.

Maintain Hobbies: Engaging in activities that patients enjoy can help reduce stress and improve their mood. Patients and caregivers should continue to pursue hobbies and activities that they find fulfilling.

Seek Professional Help: It is essential to seek professional help if patients or caregivers feel overwhelmed or depressed. Mental health professionals can provide counseling and support to help manage stress, anxiety, and depression.

Setting realistic goals: Setting small, achievable goals can help you and your caregivers feel a sense of accomplishment and improve your mood.

Being kind to yourself: It is important to acknowledge that dealing with prostate cancer is difficult and to be gentle with yourself. Don't be scared to seek for help or take time for yourself when you need it.

In conclusion, coping with prostate cancer can be challenging for both patients and their caregivers. However, with the right strategies, patients and caregivers can manage their stress and improve their quality of life. Seeking support, communication, education, healthy lifestyle, managing side effects maintaining hobbies, and seeking professional help are all essential coping strategies for patients with prostate cancer and their caregivers.

5.3 SUPPORT RESOURCES FOR PATIENTS AND FAMILIES

Prostate cancer is a serious medical condition that affects millions of people every year. For those who are diagnosed with this disease, it can be a very stressful and overwhelming time, both for the patient and their families. Fortunately, there are many support resources available to help patients and their loved ones through this difficult period. By taking advantage of these resources, patients can access the information, emotional support, and practical guidance they need to manage the disease and achieve the best possible outcome.

Some of the most helpful resources for those dealing with prostate cancer include:

Prostate Cancer Foundation: The Prostate Cancer Foundation is a nonprofit organization that provides information, support, and research funding for those affected by prostate cancer. The organization offers a range of resources, including educational materials, support groups, and a helpline that can provide guidance on treatment options and other concerns.

American Cancer Society: The American Cancer Society is a national organization that offers a wide range of support resources for cancer patients and their families. Their website provides information on prostate cancer diagnosis, treatment, and survivorship, as well as resources for emotional support and financial assistance.

Us TOO International: Us TOO International is a nonprofit organization that provides education, support, and advocacy for men and their families who are affected by prostate cancer. They offer a range of resources, including a helpline, support groups, and educational materials on treatment options and managing side effects.

National Cancer Institute: The National Cancer Institute is a government organization that provides research, education, and support resources for cancer patients and their families. Their website offers a wealth of information on prostate cancer diagnosis, treatment, and clinical trials, as well as resources for emotional support and coping with the disease.

Cancer Care: Cancer Care is a nonprofit organization that provides support services for cancer patients and their families, including counseling, financial assistance, and educational resources. They offer free counseling services over the phone, online, and in person, and can provide guidance on managing the emotional and practical challenges of living with prostate cancer.

Zero – The End of Prostate Cancer: Zero – The End of Prostate Cancer is a nonprofit organization that works to raise awareness of prostate cancer and fund research into finding a cure. They offer a range of resources, including educational materials, support groups, and advocacy programs, as well as a helpline that can provide guidance on treatment options and other concerns.

CHAPTER 6

LIVING WITH PROSTATE CANCER

The first step to living with prostate cancer is breaking the silence and speaking out about your symptoms to a healthcare provider who would carry out some tests to confirm the diagnosis. Following this is accepting the diagnosis and assessing options for treatment at the early stages. In most situations, men are ashamed to speak out when they are facing challenges with their health which is why they usually have a poor prognosis due to late presentation. It is essential that men learn to break the silence. Speak to your loved ones about your condition, their encouragement and care would help you find hope while living with this condition, and taking the necessary measures as advised by your doctor would help you take control of your health.

One prostate cancer survivor who was a teacher while talking about his journey said, ''When I was diagnosed of this condition, I didn't know how to feel or what to expect. I have heard of several people who suffered prostate cancer and didn't make it, but then, I was assured by my doctor that since it was in the early stages, something could be done. One thing I knew is that I had to do something about it. I couldn't imagine leaving my son who was just 12 and all the plans we had together. Then, my wife?, The angel that has supported me all through the years. I had to fight. Despite this diagnosis and making the choice to undergo a surgery, I also knew that I had to inform my students of my condition which has been the reason for my absence, I didn't feel ashamed expressing how I felt which I know can be hard for a lot of men. I just didn't see it as a sign of weakness but these students gave me hope which helped me through this journey. Going in for the surgery, I wasn't expectant of anything but I was sure that given a chance to live through a successful surgery would be one of life's greatest blessing to me. The surgery was successful and yes! I learnt to manage the side effects of this treatment and lived through this by follow-up care and lifestyle modifications".

6.1 MANAGING SIDE EFFECTS OF TREATMENT

In chapter 4, we discussed the various treatment options and their side effects. These side effects of prostate cancer treatment depend on the type of treatment and the patient's overall health. It can be challenging to manage and can affect your quality of life, however, you should communicate openly with your health care team about the side effects you are experiencing and follow the treatment plan. The healthcare team can provide support and guidance on managing side effects, improving the patient's quality of life.

The following are some common side effects and ways to manage them.

Urinary Incontinence: Urinary incontinence is a common side effect of prostate cancer treatment, especially after surgery or radiation therapy. It can cause embarrassment and social isolation. The patient should avoid drinking too much liquid before going to bed and practice Kegel exercises to strengthen the pelvic floor muscles. Wearing absorbent pads can also help.

Erectile Dysfunction: Erectile dysfunction is another common side effect of prostate cancer treatment, especially after surgery or radiation therapy. It can cause stress and anxiety in the patient's relationship. The patient can use oral medications like Viagra or Cialis, or use penile injections or vacuum erection devices to achieve an erection.

Fatigue: Fatigue is a common side effect of prostate cancer treatment, especially after radiation therapy or chemotherapy. The patient should get plenty of rest and exercise regularly. Consuming a balanced diet can also help to minimize fatigue.

Hot Flashes: Hot flashes are a common side effect of hormone therapy. The patient can try dressing in layers, drinking cold beverages, and avoiding spicy foods to manage hot flashes. Some medications, like antidepressants and blood pressure medication, can also help to reduce hot flashes.

Bone Loss: Hormone therapy can cause bone loss in some patients. The patient should consume a diet rich in calcium and vitamin D and take calcium and vitamin D supplements. The patient should also engage in weight-bearing exercises to maintain bone health.

6.2 FOLLOW-UP CARE AND MONITORING

After undergoing treatment for prostate cancer, it is essential for patients to continue with regular follow-up care and monitoring. This is necessary to monitor for any signs of recurrence or complications and ensure optimal recovery and health. Here are some important aspects of follow-up care and monitoring for prostate cancer patients after treatment.

PSA Tests

One of the most important aspects of follow-up care and monitoring for prostate cancer patients is monitoring their prostate-specific antigen (PSA) levels. PSA is a protein produced by the prostate gland, and elevated levels can indicate the presence of cancer or its recurrence. Patients will typically have their PSA levels checked regularly after treatment to monitor for any changes.

Physical Examinations

In addition to PSA tests, physical examinations can also be important for monitoring prostate cancer patients after treatment. During these exams, doctors will check for any signs of recurrence or complications, such as nodules or swelling in the prostate gland or surrounding tissues.

Imaging Tests

Imaging tests, such as CT scans, MRIs, and bone scans, can also be important for monitoring prostate cancer patients after treatment. These tests can help detect any signs of cancer recurrence or metastasis in other parts of the body.

Monitoring Side Effects

Prostate cancer treatments, such as surgery or radiation therapy, can sometimes cause side effects. These can include urinary incontinence, erectile dysfunction, or bowel problems. Monitoring and managing these side effects can be an important part of follow-up care and can help ensure patients' quality of life.

Psychological Support

Prostate cancer and its treatment can be emotionally challenging for patients and their families. Therefore, providing psychological support is an important aspect of follow-up care. This can include counseling, support groups, or other resources to help patients and their families cope with the emotional impact of the disease.

6.3 LIFESTYLE CHANGES AND PREVENTION STRATEGIES

Fortunately, with advances in medical technology, prostate cancer can be treated effectively. However, the treatment may have some side effects that can impact a patient's lifestyle. Here, we will explore some lifestyle changes and prevention strategies that can help patients after prostate cancer treatment. With this, patients can maintain a healthy lifestyle and reduce the risk of cancer recurrence. Patients should also talk to their healthcare provider about ways to incorporate these changes into their daily routine.

Exercise Regularly: Engaging in physical activities is one of the most effective ways to maintain a healthy lifestyle. It can also help patients recover from prostate cancer treatment. Exercise can reduce the risk of developing other medical conditions, such as heart disease, stroke, and diabetes. Additionally, it can help manage fatigue, which is a common side effect of prostate cancer treatment. Patients should aim to get at least 30 minutes of exercise a day, such as walking, swimming, or cycling.

Maintain a Healthy Diet: A healthy diet is essential for overall health and can help prevent prostate cancer recurrence. Patients should consume foods such as fruits, vegetables, whole grains, and lean protein. Additionally, they should limit their intake of red meat, processed foods, and sugary drinks. Patients should also aim to maintain a healthy weight, as obesity can increase the risk of cancer recurrence.

Quit Smoking: Smoking is a leading cause of cancer and can increase the risk of prostate cancer recurrence. Patients who smoke should desists from the habit as soon as possible. Quitting smoking can reduce the risk of developing other medical conditions, such as heart disease and lung cancer. Patients can talk to their healthcare provider about strategies to help them quit smoking.

Limit Alcohol Intake: Alcohol consumption can increase the risk of developing prostate cancer and other medical conditions. Patients should restrict their intake of alcoholic beverages to no more than one drink daily. Additionally, they should avoid binge drinking, which can increase the risk of cancer recurrence.

Manage Stress: Stress can have a negative impact on overall health and can increase the risk of cancer recurrence. Patients should find ways to manage stress, such as practicing relaxation techniques, talking to a counselor, or engaging in activities they enjoy. Patients should also get enough sleep, as lack of sleep can contribute to stress.

CHAPTER 7

FUTURE OF PROSTATE CANCER

What lies in the forthcoming years in the management and treatment of prostate cancer. With the technological advancement, would there really be a cure?. The future of prostate cancer looks brighter than ever, with exciting advances in diagnosis, treatment, and prevention. Screening and early detection, precision medicine, immunotherapy, and prevention are all promising areas of research that are shaping the future of prostate cancer. While there is still much work to be done, these innovations offer hope for a future where prostate cancer is a treatable and preventable disease. In this chapter, we will explore some of the most promising strategies and innovations that are shaping the future of prostate cancer.

7.1 ADVANCES IN RESEARCH AND TREATMENT

Over the past few decades, there have been significant advances in research and treatment for prostate cancer, leading to improved outcomes and a better quality of life for those affected by the disease. While there is still much work to be done, these innovations offer hope for a future where prostate cancer is a treatable and preventable disease.

Screening and Early Detection

One of the most promising areas of research in prostate cancer is screening and early detection. There are several new diagnostic tools and tests being developed that could greatly improve our ability to detect prostate cancer early, when it is most treatable. For example, new imaging technologies, such as multiparametric MRI, and positron emission tomography (PET) scans are providing more detailed and accurate images of the prostate, which can help doctors identify cancerous tissue earlier. This early detection is critical because it allows doctors to begin treatment sooner, when the cancer is more responsive to treatment and has not yet caused significant damage to surrounding tissues.

In addition, researchers are working on developing new blood tests that can detect prostate cancer more accurately than current tests, such as the PSA test.

Precision Medicine

Another exciting area of research in prostate cancer is precision medicine. Precision medicine is an approach to treatment that takes into account the specific genetic characteristics of an individual's tumor, allowing doctors to tailor treatment to the patient's unique needs. This approach has already shown promising results in other types of cancer, and researchers are now exploring its potential in prostate cancer. For example, there are now several targeted therapies that are designed to attack specific molecular targets in prostate cancer cells, which could offer more effective and less toxic treatment options.

Immunotherapy

Immunotherapy is another innovative approach to treating prostate cancer that is showing great promise. Immunotherapy works by harnessing the power of the immune system to target and kill cancer cells. There are several different types of immunotherapy being developed for prostate cancer, including immune checkpoint inhibitors, CAR-T cell therapy, and cancer vaccines. These therapies have already shown promising results in clinical trials, and researchers are continuing to explore their potential.

Another major area of progress in prostate cancer research has been the development of new treatment options that are more effective and less invasive than traditional treatments. For example, robotic-assisted surgery is a minimally invasive surgical technique that uses a robot to perform surgery with greater precision and control. This approach has been shown to reduce the risk of complications and speed up recovery times for patients.

In addition to surgical treatments, there have been significant advancements in radiation therapy and chemotherapy. These treatments have become more targeted and personalized, allowing doctors to tailor the treatment to the individual needs of each patient. For example, some radiation therapies use high-energy radiation to kill cancer cells, while sparing healthy tissue.

Prevention

Prevention is also a key area of focus in prostate cancer research. While there is no surefire way to prevent prostate cancer, there are several lifestyle factors that can reduce a man's risk of developing the disease. For example, maintaining a healthy weight, exercising regularly, and eating a diet rich in fruits, vegetables, and whole grains can all help reduce the risk of prostate cancer.

In addition, researchers are exploring the potential of certain drugs, such as finasteride and dutasteride, to prevent prostate cancer in men at high risk. There have also been significant advancements in the development of new drugs that can slow the progression of prostate cancer and improve outcomes for patients. For example, hormone therapy is a type of drug therapy that can slow the growth of prostate cancer by reducing the levels of testosterone in the body. Other drugs target specific proteins that are involved in the growth and spread of cancer cells, preventing them from multiplying and spreading.

Overall, the advances in research and treatment for prostate cancer have greatly improved the outlook for those diagnosed with this disease. With earlier detection, more precise treatments, and a greater understanding of the biology of the disease, patients can receive more effective and personalized care, leading to better outcomes and a better quality of life.

7.2 EMERGING THERAPIES AND TECHNOLOGIES

Prostate cancer is a complex ailment that requires an interdisciplinary approach to treatment. Several emerging therapies and technologies that can be used to treat prostate cancer such as targeted therapies, immunotherapy, radiopharmaceuticals, MRI-guided biopsy, and focal therapy have developed over time as a result of medical technology advancement and they offer new options for the treatment of prostate cancer. As research continues, it is likely that even more effective and less invasive treatments will be developed, improving the prognosis for men with this disease. In this section of

Chapter 7, we will explore some of the most promising new treatments for prostate cancer.

Targeted Therapies

Targeted therapies are a type of cancer treatment that uses drugs to target specific molecules involved in cancer growth and progression. These drugs work by interfering with the signals that cancer cells use to grow and divide, ultimately leading to the death of these cells.

Several targeted therapies have been approved for the treatment of prostate cancer, including enzalutamide, abiraterone, and apalutamide. These drugs have been shown to be effective in reducing the size of tumors and delaying disease progression in men with advanced prostate cancer.

Radiopharmaceuticals

Radiopharmaceuticals are drugs that contain a radioactive substance that can be used to kill cancer cells. These drugs are typically administered intravenously and can be targeted specifically to cancer cells, sparing healthy tissue from radiation exposure.

Several radiopharmaceuticals have been approved for the treatment of prostate cancer, including radium-223 and lutetium-177. These drugs have been shown to be effective in reducing the size of tumors and delaying disease progression in men with advanced prostate cancer.

MRI-Guided Biopsy

MRI-guided biopsy is a new technology that uses magnetic resonance imaging (MRI) to guide the placement of biopsy needles. This technology allows doctors to more accurately target suspicious areas of the prostate gland, improving the accuracy of prostate cancer diagnosis.

Focal Therapy

Focal therapy is a type of cancer treatment that targets only the areas of the prostate gland where cancer is present. This treatment can be used to treat early-stage prostate cancer and can help preserve the function of the prostate gland.

Several focal therapy techniques are currently being studied for the treatment of prostate cancer, including high-intensity focused ultrasound (HIFU) and cryotherapy.

7.3 HOPE FOR A CURE

Is there really a cure for prostate cancer?

Despite the prevalence of prostate cancer, there is reason to believe that a cure for prostate cancer may be on the horizon. In recent years, there have been significant advances in the detection, diagnosis, and treatment of this disease, giving hope to those who are affected by it.

One promising area of research involves the use of immunotherapy to treat prostate cancer which has shown great promise in clinical trials, with some patients experiencing long-term remission of their cancer. Another area is precision medicine which provides certain information about the individual's tumor genetic characteristics. This information can then be used to develop targeted therapies that are more effective at treating the cancer while minimizing side effects.

In addition to these promising treatments, there are also efforts underway to improve early detection and diagnosis of prostate cancer. New screening tests are being developed that can detect the disease at earlier stages, when it is more easily treatable. This is important because prostate cancer often grows slowly, and early detection can lead to more successful treatment outcomes.

Despite the progress that has been made, there is still much work to be done in the fight against prostate cancer. Researchers are continuing to explore new treatments and strategies for prevention, and it will likely be several years before a cure is found. However, with the continued efforts of the medical community and the support of patients and their families, there is reason to believe that a cure for prostate cancer is within reach.

If you or someone you know has been diagnosed with prostate cancer, it is important to remember that there is hope for a cure. By staying informed about the latest research and treatment options, and by working closely with your healthcare team, you can help to ensure the best possible outcome for yourself or your loved one. Together, we can work towards a future where prostate cancer is a curable disease.

CONCLUSION

Prostate cancer is one of the most common cancers affecting millions of men around the world and this usually occurs in men beyond their 50's. This condition can be quite overwhelming and challenging for the individual, however, an early detection can increase the survival rates of men with this condition.

"Prostate Cancer Unveiled" is a powerful and informative book that sheds light on a topic that affects so many men and their loved ones. It is a testament to the power of knowledge and empowerment and provides a comprehensive overview of the disease, including risk factors, diagnosis, and treatment options, while also sharing personal stories and experiences to help readers understand the emotional impact of a prostate cancer diagnosis. The stories and advice shared in this book will help those affected by prostate cancer navigate their journey with confidence and strength. It also shares the advances in the research and treatment of prostate cancer while hoping for a cure in the future. Most importantly, the book empowers men to take control of their health by encouraging them to have open conversations with their doctors, make informed decisions about their care, and prioritize self-care. Through education, awareness, and advocacy, we can break the silence surrounding prostate cancer and find hope in the fight against this disease. This book is a valuable resource for anyone impacted by prostate cancer and serves as a beacon of hope for those on the journey to recovery.

www.ingramcontent.com/pod-product-compliance
Lightning Source LLC
Chambersburg PA
CBHW071029220526
45467CB00004B/1576